THE BREATH OF
GOD OVER
ESSENTIAL OILS

L. EMERSON FERRELL

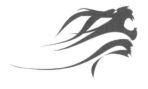

Ana Méndez Ferrell Inc.

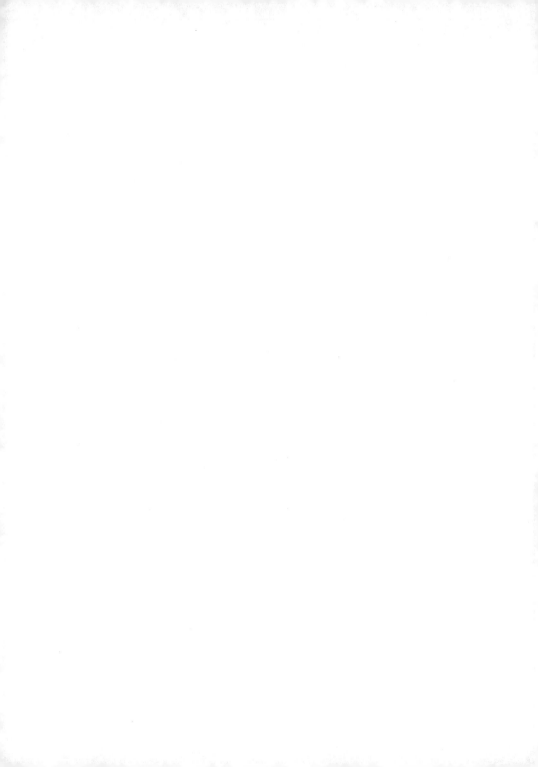

THE BREATH OF
GOD OVER
ESSENTIAL OILS

L. EMERSON FERRELL

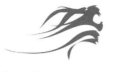

Ana Méndez Ferrell Inc.

The Breath of God, over Essential Oils

© L. EMERSON FERRELL

1ST Edition 2012.

All Scripture quotations, unless otherwise indicated, have been taken from the New King James Version.

Category: Reformation

Published by: Ana Méndez Ferrell, Inc.
                 P. O. Box 141
                 Ponte Vedra, Florida, 32004-0141
                 United States of America

Printed in: United States of America

www.AnaMendezFerrell.com

ISBN 10: 1-933163-71-2
ISBN 13: 978-1-933163-71-0

Table of Content

INTRODUCTION

A ccording to the National Association of Holistic Aromatherapy, essential oils are "highly concentrated aromatic extracts which are distilled from a variety of aromatic plant material."

Essential oils are used neat, or undiluted, as well as diluted with carrier oils and utilized for their intense fragrance as well as their therapeutic properties.

My purpose in producing Heavenly Scent Frequencies (HSF) is to provide the "Body of Christ" with a safe, effective and divine alternative to prescription medications.

Essential Oils have been used from the beginning of time. Physicians used them for centuries until cities began to flourish faster than sanitary systems could dispose of the waste from the population. The outbreak of plagues and disease forced science to create "wonder drugs" called antibiotics.

The widespread use of antibiotics has created super strains of bacteria more and more resistant to antibiotics. The drug companies are making more aggressive drugs with horrendous side affects. This forces people to take more drugs to combat the affects of the antibiotics.

The result is a society of over medicated and spiritually deprived people dependent on doctors rather than Christ. This is the condition I find people wherever I go. Deep down, they want to be free but have been trained since birth that it is ok to be a Christian and trust physicians over the cross of Christ.

The Holy Spirit explained the following to me. "Those who want to follow Christ must die in order to be resurrected. That is the process of the born again experience. Jesus was anointed for death with oils but many people don't understand the significance of that act."

I was one of those people until I studied the use of them in the scriptures. According to the book by David Stewart, Healing Oils of the Bible there are more than 500 references to essential oils in the Bible.

Essential oils are composed of hydrocarbons molecules small enough to penetrate the skin and enter directly into the blood stream with rich, powerful antioxidants. In addition they have the ability to clean and rewrite cells that have been corrupted with the poisons of medications.

Essential oils carry the consciousness of plants, which are designed to serve and heal mankind. Have you ever stood in the room of a very old home or castle and wondered what you might learn if the walls could speak? Guess what, plants have been around since creation and contain the secrets of the universe coursing through their stems and leaves.

I believe the more we use the essential oils the greater understanding we will receive of our purpose and God's love. The power of healing is transmitted in the oils because they know their creator.

The oils I create carry my relationship and revelation of Christ, which is ever increasing. The oils amplify His nature in me and combine it with His desire for all of creation.

Then it is only a matter of time before the user realizes he or she has been buried and resurrected in Christ. The process does not stop there but opens heaven for a continual interaction with the Holy Spirit.

Never let yourself become content or satisfied with the

knowledge of Christ you experience today. Each day and in everyway allow the gift of Christ to be amplified in your life. The kingdom of God is not static but ever expanding and your consciousness of Him must suffer violence if you are not reacting the same way.

1

HEAVENS SCENTS

H ave you ever been walking somewhere and suddenly smelled a fragrance that propelled you back in time to relive an event? How can aromas awaken memories inside us that recreate experiences from years ago and make them seem like they just happened? These questions are the subject of many studies in science.

Over the past several years science has discovered smell to be one of the most powerful tools for changing the attitudes and physical health of people. Although not all memories associated with smells are pleasant it, has been shown to connect the past with the present. This would seem to indicate it is possible to reshape our tomorrows from fragrances of today.

God designed that mechanism in man. After studying the scriptures I found some amazing revelation about oils, aromas and smells that opened my understanding to another dimension of our amazing Lord.

For example, there are approximately 1000 references in the Bible involving 33 species of aromatic herbs and trees. The book of Revelation says, "the leaves of the tree were for the healing of the nations."

Pharmaceutical companies use as their base compounds herbs from the plant kingdom but destroy their healing properties by changing the molecular structures, which actually poison the organism over time. Greed is the reason because governments will not issue patents on "natural" substances in nature. Thus in order to get patents chemist have to create unnatural compounds.

The following are examples of the significance of aromas in the scriptures and how they relate to man and God.

Gen. 8:21 And the LORD smelled a soothing aroma. Then the LORD said in His heart, "I will never again curse the ground for man's sake, although the imagination of man's heart is evil from his youth; nor will I again destroy every living thing as I have done.

Ex. 30:8 When Aaron sets up the lamps at twilight, he must burn incense. There is to be incense offering before the LORD throughout your generations.

Lev. 16:12 Then he shall take a censer full of burning coals of fire from the altar before the LORD, with his hands full of sweet incense beaten fine, and bring it inside the veil.

Lev. 16:13 And he shall put the incense on the fire before the LORD, that the cloud of incense may cover the mercy seat that is on the Testimony, lest he die.

Lev. 26:31 I will lay your cities waste and bring your sanctuaries to desolation, and I will not smell the fragrance of your sweet aromas.

Song 1:3 Because of the fragrance of your good ointments, Your name is ointment poured forth;

Song 1:12 While the king is at his table, My spikenard sends forth its fragrance.

John 12:3 Then Mary took a pound of very costly oil of spikenard, anointed the feet of Jesus, and wiped His feet with her hair. And the house was filled with the fragrance of the oil.

2 Cor. 2:14 But I thank God, who always leads us in victory because of Christ. Wherever we go, God uses us to make clear what it means to know Christ. It's like a fragrance that fills the air.

2 Cor. 2:15 To God we are the aroma of Christ among those who are saved and among those who are dying.

I believe those who have intimacy with Christ on a daily basis attract the aroma of His glory. In fact, on many occasions during our worship the people have smelled a fragrance filling the room. I believe the power to change our tomorrows begins with abiding in His presence today. The use of certain fragrances enhances that encounter much more than we may know.

My purpose for introducing this subject is to awaken the Body of Christ to a tool that is capable of changing their physical and mental condition.

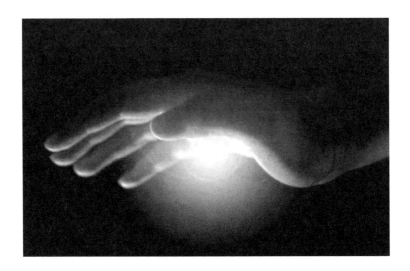

2

JESUS IS THE AROMA OF LIFE

Song 2:1 I am the rose of Sharon, and the lily of the valleys.

H ave you ever wondered why Jesus was compared with flowers?

The material world was designed and formed from the mind and voice of God who is Spirit. It only stands to reason that God would provide everything necessary to maintain His creation in the physical dimension. He knew man would depend on his senses more than His Spirit, which Adam proved in the garden. Therefore, He provided the plant kingdom with the ability to heal, deliver and even improve our spiritual attraction for Him.

In fact, while sitting outside one day listening to the birds and smelling the aroma of jasmine and orange blossoms, the Holy Spirit said, "the earth operates in perfect harmony through My aromas, sound, and light. Man is incapable of destroying that balance."

Rom. 8:19 All creation is eagerly waiting for God to reveal who his children are.

That revelation opened my understanding about the relationship between heaven and earth. The invisible world is interacting all the time with the material world in majestic ways that can be experienced in aromas, light and sound. The greater our awareness to this design the sooner our bodies and mind will respond to the groans of nature.

God never changed His command for man to *"be fruitful and multiply; fill the earth and subdue it: have dominion over the fish, birds and every living thing that moves on the earth."*

The earth is waiting to share its secrets with those who understand their responsibility of stewardship over Gods creation. But most of the Church is sick, tired, diseased and deaf to His call. God is awakening our understanding to the tools already in nature to change our sickness into health and renew our strength for the season ahead.

3
TEMPLE RESTORATION

1 Cor. 6:19 what, know ye not that your body is the temple of the Holy Spirit which is in you, which ye have from God, and ye are not your own?

The Lord has taught me over the years the importance of health in every area of our being. The battle began after my spirit was awakened in rebirth, according to the model Jesus described to Nicodemus in John 3: 3-6. He said, "you must be born of the water and Spirit to see the kingdom of God." Read my book *Immersed In Him* for a deeper revelation of those words.

The soul is the most resistant to change. It is the center for emotions, thoughts and beliefs. Most people make their decisions in life based on the assumption that the physical world is "the" only reality. Therefore, each person spends their formative years defining who they are and what they believe from their surroundings and culture.

Most of the population in the western world derives their opinions and beliefs from the material world. So, it would make sense that the majority of the Church are raised to believe consulting a physician for physical and psychological disorders are acceptable to Christ.

However, if that were true then the death and resurrection of Christ was only partially redeeming. Wait a minute; Jesus said on the cross "it is finished," and what about the scriptures in Isaiah and Peter that describe His wounds and stripes were for our healing? (Isaiah 53:5, Peter 2:24)

Changing what we believe as Christians is the key to entering divine health. Unfortunately, wrong beliefs have contributed to the majority of Christians neglecting their temples.

If God's Spirit is not governing our soul and body, our physical temple will be in disarray, which hinders the Holy Spirit from ministering health to our bodies and mind.

My greatest experiences with the Holy Spirit are the result of changing the way I perceive Him. That opens my heart and mind to eternity. This happens over and over again in our times of worship, which incidentally releases corporate faith for outstanding miracles.

Often the Lord heals people, in order for them to focus on Him and His goodness. It is during these times the tangible presence of God can be felt and no words can describe the healing that transpires in their minds and bodies. I believe if we can maintain this environment in our daily lives our temples or physical bodies will experience the supernatural more often.

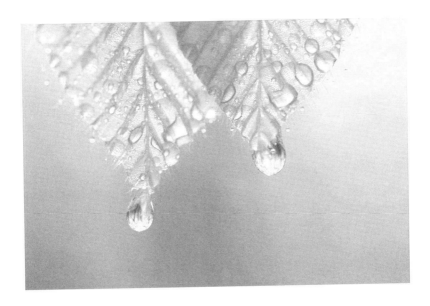

4

ESSENTIAL OILS AS FREQUENCY

M any Christians may resist essential oils because of a *new age* connotation toward the term aromatherapy. Some think oils are to be used only for anointing purposes by priests or pastors. Many ministers consider the anointing oil as symbolic only, and do not recognize their therapeutic value. But as the scriptures reveal, God was the one who loved aromas and made them an integral part of creation.

Of the five senses, smell is the most sensitive to awaken the spiritual nature of man. Aromas, mixed with light and sound impact the brain in unusual ways outside of reason, and can produce total healing in the soul and body.

For example, the molecular weight of essential oils is small enough to penetrate human skin, cells of the lungs and straight to the brain. These messengers of health carry cellular intelligence at the level of DNA.

Moreover, when you inhale oil molecules they are detected by the brain olfactory center, which stimulates the central part of the called the *amygdala,* which is the processing area for emotions such as fear, anger and pleasure.

The *amygdala* is also responsible for determining what and where memories are stored in the brain. Research has shown this part of the brain reacts to smells only. It will not store words or sounds only fragrances.

Essential oils can release childhood memories and repressed emotions that may have hindered our development in Christ. The oils can act to remove toxins from our memory the same way the body removes harmful toxins from our blood.

Most people rarely deal with deep-rooted, repressed emotional traumas that can produce chemical properties that attack the immune system. For example, the stomach may produce ulcers or the kidneys create stones as a result of emotional traumas.

Physical alignments are spiritual in nature and therapeutic grade oils have the ability to open the spirit to the healing nature of our Lord.

WHY ESSENTIAL OILS ARE SO EFFECTIVE

The properties of essential oils are unique for many reasons but one of the most important feature is that they carry specific frequencies that are capable of correcting damaged cells in our bodies.

All physical matter is energy formed from atoms, which are types of electrical fields. The human body has trillions of cells that are tiny batteries designed to keep our organs functioning correctly.

If the batteries are not recharged they die creating disease in the organs. Healthy cells are the source for a strong immune system and physical well being.

Essential oils are frequencies of energy designed to recharge our cells. They are capable of cleaning and rewriting corrupted cells. Furthermore, many of the oils carry oxygen, which destroys all forms of cancer and bacteria.

Bruce Tainio measured the frequency of organs and essential oils. Though the precise numbers may vary, the following frequency charts for both organs and essential oils have been accepted as a general guideline.

ORGANS	FREQUENCIES
Brain frequency indicates a genius	80-82 MHz,
Healthy body (neck down)	62-68 MHz
Thyroid and Parathyroid glands	62-68 MHz
Thymus Gland	65-68MHz
Heart	67-70 MHz
Lungs	58-65MHz
Liver	55-65MHz
Pancreas	60-80 MHz
Stomach	58-65 MHz
Ascending Colon	58-60 MHz

ORGANS	FREQUENCIES
Descending Colon	58-63 MHz
Disease begins (ie. Colds)	59-60 MHz
Flu like symptoms	58 MHz
Viral Infection	55 MHz
Epstein Barr	52 MHz
Tissue breakdown from disease	48 MHz
Cancer	42 MHz
Death begins	20 MHz

Observe the vibrational frequencies operating in essential oils.

ESSENTIAL OILS   FREQUENCIES

ESSENTIAL OILS	FREQUENCIES
Rose (Rosa damascene)	320 MHz
Helichrysum	181 MHz
Frankincense	147 MHz
Ravintsara	134MHz
Lavender (Lavendula angustifolia)	118 MHz
Myrrh (Commiphora myrrha)	105 MHz
Blue Chamomile (Matricaria recutita)	105 MHz
Melissa	102 MHz
Sandalwood (Santalum album)	96 MHz
Peppermint (Mentha peperita)	78 MHz

A healthy person radiates a cellular frequency between 62-68 MHZ. If the cell decreases to 58 MHZ, cold and flu symptoms are likely to arise.

Candida starts at 55 MHZ (*Candida albicans is a type of yeast or a fungus that is found in the body. Having these bacteria inside the body is healthy but when there is too much of this, infections or disease may occur*)

Epstein Barr breeds at 52 MHZ (*a common human virus that causes infectious mononucleosis* and plays a role in the emergence of two rare forms of cancer: Burkitt's *lymphoma,* and nasopharyngeal carcinoma).

Cancer begins just below 42 MHZ while cell decomposition to death begins at 25 MHZ.

The measured frequencies of essential oils begin at 52 MHz, and go as high as 320 MHz.

For comparison, fresh produce has a frequency up to 15 MHz, dry herbs from 12 to 22 MHz, and fresh herbs from 20 to 27 MHz. Processed and canned foods have no measurable frequency whatsoever.

Research shows that essential oils have the highest frequencies of any natural substance known to man, creating an environment in which diseases such as bacteria, virus, fungi and so on, cannot exist. Essential oils are said to align frequencies, thus balancing and harmonizing body organs.

Blending essential oils can amplify frequencies, and this amplification is sometimes referred to as **synergy.** Essential oils are multifunctional, giving them a wide range of use.

They are absorbed into the bloodstream within seconds of application and stay in a healthy body for up to eight hours. Adding heat to the application site produces faster penetration and results.[1]

---

[1] Stewart, David (2002) <u>Healing Oils of The Bible,</u> Care Publications, Marble Hill, MO. 32-34 pp

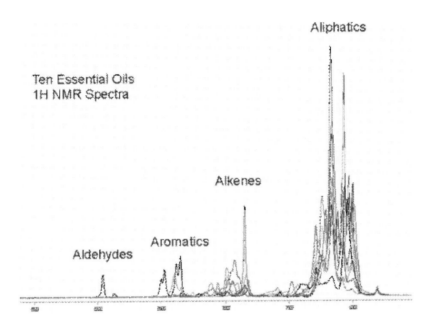

5
CREATE HEALTHY CELLS

D r Robert O. Becker, in his book *The Body Electric*, tells us the human body has an electrical frequency, and its frequency levels can determine much about a person's health.

I think it is important to understand essential oils from both a spiritual and scientific point of view. The research on oils and their affect on human beings is astounding.

As already mentioned the physical world is composed of atoms. Every atom in the universe has a specific vibratory or periodic motion.

Each periodic motion has a frequency that can be measured in Hertz. Every element in the Periodic Table has a specific vibrational frequency. The frequency of a current is measured in Hertz. A hertz is one revolution from one point to another.

For example, if you dropped a rock in a puddle of water the wave emanating from that splash to a defined point and back to the impact point is considered a revolution. A 100-watt electric light bulb operating at 60htz means it blinks on and off 60 times a second.

Voltage and frequency are important for understanding the way human cells operate. Voltage is described as the power to do work, while the movement of electrons is measured in amperage.

Increasing the voltage causes electrons to move faster thereby creating a vortex or concentric circles. A magnetic field is created by and around the vortex.

The magnetic field and amperage are related to the frequency produced by the electrons. The faster the electrons move the greater the magnetic field and higher the frequency.

Our bodies are composed of trillions of cells that are formed from atoms vibrating at a wide range of frequencies. These cells require voltage and frequency to operate at maximum conditions. Disease occurs when the cells have too little voltage and are running at too low a frequency.

When disease and illness are present, they may manifest as chemical imbalances. That generally means an electromagnetic imbalance has altered the specific vibrational frequencies of molecules, cells, tissues and organs within the body.

Our organs are created to support each other in perfect rhythm, but when disease disrupts that harmony, illness such as cancer, heart attacks, and diabetes are the result.

"Resetting" the body to its original frequency brings it into balance and restores its natural harmonic resonance, which corrects the cells corruption from disease.

The body is created with trillions of microorganisms designed to decompose the body after death. These bugs remain dormant as long as the frequencies of the cells operate above 52 MHz. This requires the proper nutrients such as oxygen, water and exercise to name a few. If the microorganisms awake because of harmonic dissonance or low voltage they release enzymes to dissolve the cells for food.

For example, if cells in the throat loses enough voltage they will awaken bacteria called streptococcus. This feels like an itchy, sore throat. This usually provokes a visit to the doctor who generally prescribes an antibiotic[2] that does not kill the bacteria but usually alleviates the symptoms.

Unfortunately, antibiotics are designed to treat a symptom and further lower the frequency of the organism, which eventually produces chronic diseases in the body.

---

[2] Tennant, Jerry (2010) Healing is Voltage, Made in U.S.A. Lexington, KY. 60-61 ppg.

When you inhale or apply essential oils, you are in effect cleaning and reprogramming the cells in order for them to repair the body. This simple act mixed with faith will allow the Holy Spirit to heal our bodies and bring peace to our souls.

God designed our bodies to heal themselves perpetually through healthy reproduction of new cells. Our blood is the primary source of this healing nature. The blood was created by God and designed to reproduce healthy cells in every human being. Sin corrupted the spiritual nature of man and thus is the source for all sickness and disease.

That is why all sickness is spiritual and until it is dealt with at that level will pass from generation to generation. Science likes to call sickness and disease that goes from family to family "genetics." The truth is if you want your future generation to be free from sickness change your spiritual DNA. That is accomplished with a blood transfusion with The Son of God, Christ Jesus.

Essential oils are not a substitute for the Holy Spirit and The Cross of Christ but are a divine tool used throughout scriptures to facilitate the healing power of God. (James 5:14)

When you inhale or apply essential oils, you are in effect cleaning and reprogramming the cells in order for them to repair the body. This simple act mixed with faith will allow the Holy Spirit to heal our bodies and bring peace to our souls. I believe the best strategy for divine health is prayer and fasting. But most of the Body of Christ is in critical condition from wrong choices and beliefs that require immediate attention. That is why understanding the importance of our cells, as the fundamental key to physical vitality is the first step to fulfilling our destiny in God.

The chronic illness in many of the Body of Christ has prevented it from understanding the spirit realm. Unless one is at peace with both the physical and spiritual world, the Holy Spirit will be restricted in revealing the mysteries of His Kingdom. That is why fasting has been such an integral part of my life.

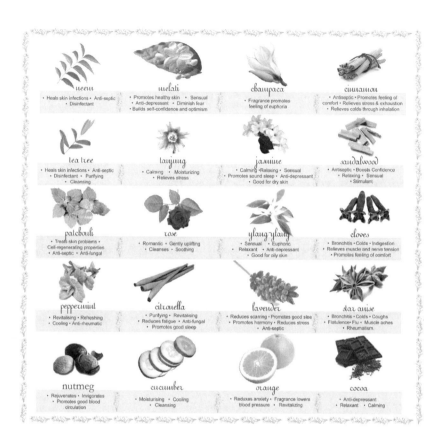

neem
- Heals skin infections • Anti-septic
- Disinfectant

melati
- Promotes healthy skin • Sensual
- Anti-depressant • Diminish fear
- Builds self-confidence and optimism

champaca
- Fragrance promotes feeling of euphoria

cinnamon
- Antiseptic • Promotes feeling of comfort • Relieves stress & exhaustion
- Relieves colds through inhalation

tea tree
- Heals skin infections • Anti-septic
- Disinfectant • Purifying
- Cleansing

tanjung
- Calming • Moisturizing
- Relieves stress

jasmine
- Calming • Relaxing • Sensual
- Promotes sound sleep • Anti-depressant
- Good for dry skin

sandalwood
- Antiseptic • Boosts Confidence
- Relaxing • Sensual
- Stimulant

patchouli
- Treats skin problems •
- Cell-regenerating properties
- Anti-septic • Anti-fungal

rose
- Romantic • Gently uplifting
- Cleanses • Soothing

ylang ylang
- Sensual • Euphoric
- Relaxant • Anti-depressant
- Good for oily skin

cloves
- Bronchitis • Colds • Indigestion
- Relieves muscle and nerve tension
- Promotes feeling of comfort

peppermint
- Revitalising • Refreshing
- Cooling • Anti-rheumatic

citronella
- Purifying • Revitalising
- Reduces fatigue • Anti-fungal
- Promotes good sleep

lavender
- Reduces scarring • Promotes good slee
- Promotes harmony • Reduces stress
- Anti-septic

star anise
- Bronchitis • Colds • Coughs
- Flatulence Flu • Muscle aches
- Rheumatism.

nutmeg
- Rejuvenates • Invigorates
- Promotes good blood circulation

cucumber
- Moisturising • Cooling
- Cleansing

orange
- Reduxes anxiety • Fragrance lowers blood pressure • Revitalizing

cocoa
- Anti-depressant
- Relaxant • Calming

6

HEAVEN SCENT FREQUENCIES AND HEALING

A. THE QUANTUM WORLD AND OILS

M y life completely changed after being born of the *water and Spirit.* Following that experience God gave me a thirst for the supernatural and His Spirit. The adventures with the Holy Spirit are to wondrous for words and have driven me to study quantum physics, in an attempt to explain some of the experiences.

Quantum physics is the closest discipline in the material world that writes about faith without actually using the word. Science recognizes dimensions beyond the subatomic view operate under different laws. The quantum world reacts to the consciousness of the observer and ultimately produces the results believed by the person or persons conducting the experiments.

The vibrational frequencies of the universe, in my opinion, are the sounds of the angelic choir worshipping Christ.

The glory released from the invisible voice of God created all the elements of the material world. Those elements are the subject of mathematicians, scientist, chemist and biologist throughout the world.

Suffice it to say the elements of hydrogen, oxygen and carbon are the primary building blocks of material life. The interaction between these elements holds the secrets between the visible and invisible world.

Carbon is the basic building block of all life, especially man. All of our hormones, enzymes, proteins, blood and DNA are primarily carbon compounds. Essential oils are 80% carbon by weight. The relationship between plants and man are much greater than photosynthesis.

The aromas created from essential oils are carbon compounds. Moreover, their molecular versatility allows them to penetrate the blood and brain of our cellular structure.

After six carbon atoms join with six atoms of hydrogen that compound is no longer considered matter but rather acts like a wave of energy with all the possibilities existing to the person experiencing the scent or aroma of the oil.

This is the realm of quantum mechanics. There are no longer absolutes only probabilities. It is the world of uncertainty. In effect, these hydrocarbon compounds are

nature's doors to the realm of the Spirit, where all things are possible if YOU can BELIEVE. In other words, what a person believes is what they will discover in the end. I believe Jesus said it best when He said, *"IF YOU CAN BELIEVE ALL THINGS ARE POSSIBLE."* The question man is held accountable for is, what and who to believe?

The answers to those questions are complicated because of religion. Nevertheless, most of us begin that way and if we persevere we will discover The Truth in the person of Christ.

Once we pass from death unto life, our spirit will connect with The Spirit and see the kingdom of God. That journey will take eternity and requires retraining the way we think and feel.

B. DANGERS OF PHARMECEUTICALS

Man has used the plant kingdom for its drugs and remedies for centuries. The advancement of science has created "wonder" drugs to combat diseases and relieve suffering throughout the world.

There is no doubt doctors have been used by God to save lives through medications. The problem is they believe the drug saved people instead of the mercy of God. Everyone should know drugs don't heal, God does.

The proliferation of prescriptions drugs has produced

horrendous conditions in society. In the United States one person in three dies of cancer, one in three suffers from allergies, one in ten will have ulcers and one in five is mentally ill. One out of five pregnancies ends in miscarriage and one quarter of a million infants are born with birth defects each year.

Today chronic illness afflicts nearly half of all Americans and causes three out of four deaths in the United States alone.

In addition the citizens of America spend one dollar out of every fourteen for medical services that is 800 billion yearly, which is more than the national deficit and the profits of all U.S. corporations combined. Less people live beyond 70 years of age than 20 years ago.[3]

It is safe to say, science and medicine have no solutions for the epidemic of illness in the United States. Many professional people believe the proliferation of antibiotics is responsible for the explosion of Alzheimer's, diabetes, epilepsy and autism.

The American Cancer Society is reluctant to invest monies in genuine research through natural cures for cancer because many remedies already exist and have been proven to be

---

[3] Fallon, Sally (2001) <u>Nourishing Traditions,</u> New Trends Publishing, Inc. Washington D.C. introduction

effective. They would rather promote the belief such cures do not exist. This position allows for huge salaries and monies for "research."

Drug companies follow the same model and spend most of their money on lobbying for more funding, while creating a drug dependents society.

They will not invest in herbs and essential oils because no one can patent what is natural.

The way to big profits in the pharmaceutical industry is to create an unnatural substance that never existed before in nature, then patent it, and obtain a monopoly.

The molecules of pharmaceutical drugs are foreign to the human body.

Drugs are designed to send misinformation to cells or to block certain receptor sites in order to trick the body into giving up symptoms.

But drugs never deal with the actual disease. While they may give temporary relief to one organ they will eventually corrupt other organs.[4]

---

[4] Stewart, David, (2005). <u>The Chemistry of essential oils made simple: God's love manifest in molecules,</u> Care Publications, Marble Hill, MO pgs. 417-419

C. CHRIST IS THE CURE

We are all raised as children to trust doctors and medicine for any illness. It is time to change that belief system and trust the one who created you. He has provided a solution for every possible situation we could face in this life.

The power of Christ goes far beyond our limited understanding and initial meeting with Him.

The work of the cross was an historical fact but its authority and power is timeless. The physical dimension should not control the life of Christians. Eternity is now regardless of your surroundings.

If you believe you must wait until you physically die to live then you have never met Christ.

Jesus spoke spiritual words (John 6:63) He said, *"it is finished."* In my mind that means evil in every aspect was defeated, sickness, disease and even death were destroyed for those who BELIEVE HIM. (John 8:51, 5:24-25, 10:10)

The Bible must be read without preconceived ideas and doctrines in order to allow the Holy Spirit to retrain the way we think. That is why I believe we need our bodies and mind bathed in the frequencies of heaven.

The oils from the plants and tress processed properly can

physically reduce symptoms of disease. And when used with prayer they are capable of healing both body and soul.

The condition of most people is such that without experiencing an atmosphere charged with faith, most will make decisions from fear.

We have already discussed the frequencies associated with our bodily organs and those of therapeutic grade essential oils.

The science of quantum physics is helpful in trying to explain the mysterious interaction between our cells and essential oils.

The harmony and balance between the seen and unseen world are separated by frequencies of light.

Our human bodies are designed to be in tune with our spirit that operates according to the vibration of Christ in our lives. God created every person with an assignment and frequency that He alone controls by His will.

For example, have you noticed how easy it is to identify your voice or that of a loved one from a recording? Science calls that "voice printing" and security officials use the technology for identifying their employees.

God spoke the material world into existence and in so

doing released the full spectrum of frequencies measurable and immeasurable.

The following verse in Colossians gives us an idea of the magnitude of who and what Christ did for us before the foundation of the world.

> _Col.1:16_ For in Him was created the universe of things in heaven and on earth, things seen and things unseen, thrones, dominions, princedoms, powers—all were created, and exist through and for Him. And HE IS before all things and in and through Him the universe is a harmonious whole.

The voice of Christ is the resonant vibration that holds all things together. Not only that but His voice is the energy that forms and changes matter.

Remember when He told His disciples you should be able to speak to the mountain and tell it to go into the ocean? (Paraphrasing Matthew 17:20)

I believe Jesus is explaining the power of faith in knowing the sound of His voice as the creator of all things. It is that voice that is heard by His sheep and follows Him through the quantum world of uncertainty.

There is such a thing in science called resonance. Resonance occurs when two things vibrate in unison at the same principal frequency or frequencies.

For example, striking a tuning fork with a pitch of C will only resonate with other tuning forks of the same pitch. Many opera singers have shattered glass because they matched the tone of the crystal goblets to the pitch of their voices.

Essential oils resonate at the fundamental frequencies of our organs, tissues and cells. **Oil molecules are predesigned by Christ to sing at the right frequency for our body to resonate at His voice.**

The perfect order of all things resides in the love frequency of Christ who causes all things to live.

D. PLANTS COMMUNICATE

Plants are living breathing complex life forms with consciousness, and are as complex as the human body. There are countless studies demonstrating this fact.

Frank Loehr in his book *The Power of Prayer on Plants* demonstrated scientifically that prayer made a difference in the speed in which corn seeds germinated, grew and produced. Moreover, that prayer was not a state of mind but as real as sunlight in producing results.[5]

Another scientist by the name of Cleve Backster used

---

[5] Loehr, Franklin, (1969) The Power of Prayer on Plants, Signet Books, New York. 127 pp.

his background in lie detection to measure the response of plants, to his thoughts. In one experiment he poured hot coffee on the plant and cut its leaves. The plant responded dramatically according to the readings of his machine.

The next day he came to the room and even when he thought about doing the same thing the plant reacted. The next day he came into the room and only pretended to repeat the act but the plant read his intentions and did not react.

Furthermore, after the leaves were separated from the plants and shredded they still demonstrated the response as if they were still attached to the whole plant. This was proof the plants remain conscious in every cell of its structure including the oils.

Backster concluded that the awareness of plants extends beyond the physical dimensions of time and space. He believed they were connected to a larger whole that enabled it to respond to stimuli at a distance. That stimulus is a person named Jesus Christ.

One person by the name of Marcel Vogel attempted to replicate Backster's experiment in a class setting. He discovered, the students who did not believe it was possible, were unable to duplicate it, while those who believed, found that the plants responded accordingly.

Vogel concluded that the consciousness of the

experimenter was as much of the research as the results. This is why the world of quantum physics best describes the behavior of essential oils.[6]

A Japanese professor by the name of Masaru Emoto took vials of water and either by sending thoughts or taping words to the bottles froze them and then photographed the crystals. He found that the crystals represented the words whether audibly or by thought. Words such as angel, love, thank you, beautiful etc. produced beautiful geometric crystals. Words such as hate, fool, devil produced ugly, deformed crystals.[7]

A Swiss researcher by the name of Hans Jenny placed various finely divided powder on a surface and then submitted that surface to mechanical vibrations produced by sound.

He carefully controlled the frequencies and recorded the results with both a still and video camera. The results were fascinating in that he was able to show lifeless matter in the form of powder can be transformed into majestic forms that appear full of life just from vibrations.[8]

---

[6] Stewart, David, (2002)The Chemistry of essential oils made simple: God's love manifest in molecules, Care Publications, Marble, MO. pg.723-725

[7] Emoto, Masuru (2003) Messages from Water Hado publishing, Amstel, Amsterdam, The Netherlands 147 pp

[8] Jenny, Hans (2001) Cymatics, MACROmedia, Newmarket, New Hampshire, 295pp

If plants, water and powder respond to thought and vibrations what about essential oils? Absolutely, yes is the answer. The molecules of oil receive and transmit thoughts. They do this because God created all life to communicate His love to one another.

This means plants have consciousness and vibrate at frequencies above sin, sickness and disease. You do not have to wait for science to prove it, believe it now and experience the results.

The power to change your tomorrow will not arise from yesterday's knowledge and beliefs. The essential oils are an instrument of God to help us hear His voice of love.

7

TRUST GOD NOT DOCTORS OR MEDICINE

A. UNDERSTAND OUR CHOICES

T he word "doctor" is mentioned three times in the entire Bible (Luke 2:46, 5:17 & Acts 5:34) and is never used to indicate a healer or a medical practitioner in the modern sense of the word, but is used to mean a teacher, rabbi, or doctor of the law.

However, a doctor of the law in biblical times was also a teacher of biblical health principles. In addition, since the times of the Levitical law they were schooled in the area of health quite extensively. This is the root of holistic health, herbology, and naturopathy.

The word naturopathy means: a system of disease treatment using natural foods, light, warmth, massage, fresh air, regular exercise, and the avoidance of drugs.

The prophet Jeremiah carried a stern message from the LORD to the tribe of Judah during their days of rebellion that can also be tied in to our times with modern medicine and disease.

"Thus said the LORD; Cursed be the man that trusts in man, and makes flesh his arm (and whose heart departs from the LORD." (Jeremiah 17:5)

Another biblical example is found in mark 5:25-34 and Luke 8:43-48. These passages deal with a woman who gave all her money to doctors and yet continued to get worse.

According to these passages, a certain woman, which had an issue of blood for 12 years and had suffered many things of many physicians and spent all that she had and grew worse.

There is an important lesson to be learned that is applicable to us today. When afflicted with disease, some will ask for prayer and even confess healing with their lips, but their true faith is in physicians and hospitals.

Believing doctors over God is a deadly mistake witnessed by millions of deaths a year caused by pharmaceuticals, doctors and hospitals *(iatrogenic deaths, nosocomial infections, pharmaceutical side-effects, etc.).*

The worship of science and their medical deities must stop for all those who name Christ as their Lord or they will suffer the same as those who want nothing to do with our Christ.[9]

The original design of God was for man to understand his relationship with his Creator first. Healing and health are the byproduct of those who submit to Christ and His Word.

Physicians are for those who do not submit to Christ.

B. THE POWER OF ESSENTIAL OILS

The powers of essential oils are the result of God's intelligent design. Essential oils are likened to fine wines. Even when harvested from the same fields, variables such as rain, wind, temperature, sunlight and topsoil make them unique in consistency, purity and therapeutic values.

God knew that sin would create disease, stress and death in the world. Christ is the answer for sin, sickness and disease.

The plant kingdom works in harmony with His completed work to provide confirmation of God's glory throughout the earth.

Man relies on his limited understanding, greed and pride to produce antibiotics to fight the bacteria that his sin has produced.

---

[9] Young, D. Gary (2000) Science and Application of Essential Oils, Level I and II, YELO, Payton, Utah. 200-225 pages.

The result will be that diseases learn to recognize and adapt to man's antibiotics and drugs. That is because the synthetic drug removes the active ingredient in the plant in order to mass-produce them.

Man and pharmaceutical companies cannot wait on nature to produce the crops with the right compounds in nature to fight the diseases.

With the natural antibiotic properties of God's healing oils and built in intelligence and variability, bacteria can never anticipate ways to resist essential oils because of multiple species within each oil, potency differences and adaptability.

This assures their effectiveness will never diminish, even thousands of years later. When we apply oils our cells and organs come out stronger, our beneficial bacteria is enhanced and our immune system is strengthened not weakened.

The molecular structure of an essential oil is so small that one-drop contains enough molecules to cover all 9 trillion cells in our bodies.

Each cell has a receptor or door that opens to receives the information from the molecule. That information can change the DNA of corrupted cells and reprogram it to the right frequency designed to harmonize with the rest of our organism.

C. THE SCIENCE OF OILS

All essential oils are organic compounds composed of 5 carbon atoms with 8 hydrogen atoms attached to an oxygen molecule. They are classified under three categories- PMS.

(P) Phenylpropanoids; which clean the cell receptor sites allowing proper transfer of hormones, neurotransmitters (electrical charge) for cell communication, and energy transfer.

(M) Monoterpenes; 2,000 varieties that reprogram miswritten information in the DNA's cellular memory bank.

(S) Sesquiterpenes; 10,000 varieties that deliver oxygen molecules to brain cells and can also erase or deprogram miswritten codes of DNA. In effect floods them with oxygen and deprograms the mutated DNA.

The combination of Phenylpropanoids, Monoterpenes, and Sesquiterpenes (PMS) in blended oils has the potential to prevent and reverse almost every disease condition plaguing America.

The American Medical Association admits if they could find a drug that could penetrate the "blood brain barrier it would be the cure all." Essential oils are the answer they are looking for but it is not the one they want.

The reason they refuse to study the effects of essential oils is because of money. Healing with oils collides with the medical system in the United States and the pharmaceutical industry. There is no profit in what cannot be legally patented.

The sad truth is aromatherapy originated as a medical therapy based on the pharmacological effects of essential oils, which were considered equally effective as the conventional pharmaceutical drugs.

8

ESSENTIAL OILS AND RESTORATION

E ssential oils are to the cells what hydrogen is to water. The plant kingdom holds the keys to rejuvenation physically, emotionally and spiritually.

For example, the leaves of trees and plants do not appear old or worn unless diseased or transitioning from death to life according to the seasons.

The blood that supplies our life force is akin to the liquid that flows through the plants. The biggest differences are plants do not have wrong thoughts or consume harmful drugs and foods.

The resurrection of plants is the miracle power that is released into our bodies each time we use their oil. It is that regeneration that transforms our cells and produces anti aging antibodies inside our molecules.

Beauty products produced by cosmetic manufactures lack the scientific sophistication or the financial resources to produce the molecular compounds of essential oils. Their products are incapable of changing the DNA of corrupted cells.

The result is cosmetics that cover the skin but unable to slow the aging process. Hence, more and more people are paying for expensive cosmetic surgery procedures.

Esther of the Old Testament is a picture of the amazing power of oils both physically and mentally. The scriptures describe her bathing in Myrrh for six months. (Esther 2:12)

Myrrh vibrates at an average frequency of 105 MhZ according to research done by Bruce Tainio. It is has been my experience that oils with frequencies 90 MhZ and higher increase my desire to worship Christ. My mind and heart overflow with thanksgiving and joy. The knowledge of His presence is front and center in my thoughts.

I believe Esther was immersed in the presence of God on a daily basis for 6 months because of the Myrrh. This process beautified her skin and altered her consciousness about life, death and destiny.

The scriptures reveal her courage and resolve to deliver her people even if meant sacrificing her own life. (Esther 4-5)

God placed man in a garden surrounded by the smells and frequency of heaven. Trees and plants are not restricted by time. I believe those who touch the essence of plants by using the oils are entering the doorway to the realms of eternity.

9
MY ASSIGNMENT FOR THE BODY

O ver the years of ministry my heart has been broken by the condition of Gods people. Regardless of the places we go many of the precious people of God are suffering from sickness, disease and obesity.

> _Jam. 5:14 Is any one ill? Let him send for the Elders of the Church, and let them pray over him, after anointing him with oil in the name of the Lord._

This scripture illustrates the power of oil in combination with the prayers of believers. This is truly heaven and earth connecting through God's design for His Body.

During prayer the Lord would not let me rest until I studied the scriptures concerning oils. To say I was shocked is an understatement.

After considerable prayer and meditation the Lord compelled me to read and reread the following verses in Matthew.

It is important to understand the majority of the time the Bible is speaking about essential oils as illustrated below.

Matt. 26:11-15 A woman came to Him with a jar of very costly, sweet-scented ointment, which she poured over His head as He reclined at table. In pouring this ointment over me, her object was to prepare me for burial.

In solemn truth I tell you that wherever in the whole world this Good News shall be proclaimed, this deed of hers shall be spoken of in memory of her."

At that time one of the Twelve, the one called Judas Iscariot, went to the High Priests and said, "What are you willing to give me if I betray him to you?" So they weighed out to him thirty shekels,

Have you ever noticed the way Judas responded to that event? I believe the fragrances of heaven can make demons manifest inside of people and expose that person to the devil they may be serving. In this instance it is clear Judas was serving Mammon.

There is an interesting story in Mark that may open your eyes (no pun intended) to our connection with all of God's creation.

Mark 8:22-26 And they came to Bethsaida. And a blind man was brought to Jesus and they entreated Him to

touch him.
So He took the blind man by the arm and brought him out
of the village, and spitting into his eyes He put His hands
on him and asked him, "Can you see anything?"

He looked up and said, "I can see the people: I see them
like trees—only walking." Then for the second time He
put His hands on the man's eyes, and the man, looking
steadily, recovered his sight and saw everything distinctly.

So He sent him home, and added, "Do not even go into
the village."

I have heard many ministers say that even Jesus had to pray twice for this man to receive his sight. I don't think that is the case. I believe Jesus restored both his spiritual and physical sight.

Imagine the frequency and aroma of the Son of God's saliva penetrating the occipital lobe? That is the part of the brain that interprets what the eyes are seeing.

In my opinion, Jesus was allowing this man to see the kingdom mysteries in the earth before the foundation of the world.

Jesus opened both his spiritual and natural eyes. The man saw the heavenly dimension and could only describe it as "walking trees."

Jesus needed to remove the man from his surroundings, in order for him to see the wonders of The Kingdom. Notice Jesus instructs this man NOT to return to the village. The multiplication of God's Kingdom is hindered in places of nonbelief.

As we spoke about earlier, cell structure of essential oils' is very similar to the human cells. The essential oil of a plant and the human blood share several common properties. The primary elements in both human beings and essential oils are carbon hydrogen nitrogen oxygen.

This shared chemistry makes essential oils a powerful defense against the common afflictions of the human body. The essential oils possess potent antibacterial, anti-fungal, and antiviral properties.

Essential oils originate from the liquid in plants and are their life force the same way blood is ours. They are volatile liquids distilled from various parts of plants, including seeds, bark, leafs, stems, roots, flowers and fruit.

If a leaf or any part of a plant has been cut or damaged for some reason, the plant releases a liquid substance that protects it from further damage from microbes, bacteria, and viruses, and helps the plant to regenerate itself.

This liquid is the essential oil that helps the plant to survive, which is why essential oils are called essential.

First and foremost God is the healer. Nothing is a substitute for the Holy Spirit. Only God produces the oils that can bring healing. But if we are unable to hear His voice or abide by His word we will perish. (Hosea 4:6)

HOLY GHOST ASSIGNMENT

The Holy Ghost gave me specific instructions to prepare oils for His Body on earth with the same passion Mary anointed Him before His death. My commitment is to find the purest ingredients of God's creation to anoint His Body to restore their sight and passion for the King. God has put in my heart to create a line of essential oils called, HEAVEN SCENT FREQUENCIES.

As noted earlier most of the essential oils marketed in the world are not therapeutical quality.

Each of the oils I blend will originate from organically grown or wild crafted plants. Thus they will be formed from the highest quality and therapeutic grade materials.

After a person begins using the oils often and generously they will notice an immediate change in attitude and appetite. The spiritual power of therapeutic oils begins subtly but increase over time. (Read the section on application)

Through the wisdom and guidance of the Holy Spirit I am blending frequencies together to form the most powerful oils possible as a tool to anoint God's Body.

I believe if our physical bodies can be reset to God's factory conditions, void from chronic pain, they can receive the power of Christ and His peace that passes understanding.

The souls of so many people are trapped by emotions and thoughts created from chaos and turmoil on the inside. My goal is to be an instrument to speak to the tempest inside your bodies by applying heavens frequencies.

I believe over time people will break the chains of pain and wrong thinking and their soul will ascend to the rulership meant for His sons.

The power to rule and reign has been available to His Body for over two thousand years but for one reason or another we have found ourselves in a physical condition that has affected our ability to see and believe this truth. But God has not forsaken us or left us desolate.

I believe the Lord will give me several formulas to address the most common problems in the Body of Christ. Most people are overweight, anxious, and fearful. In addition the population in general suffers from a short attention span, weak immune systems and fatigue.

The different blends will combat many of these issues, but the oil is only a tool for a person's recovery. Once people understand they are His temples they must change their wrong eating and drinking habits. People must stop drinking soft drinks. Did you know a person gains 1 pound a month by consuming these sugar loaded drink a day? That is 12 pounds a year and 60 pounds over 5 years.

In addition people must understand and practice a lifestyle of fasting.

I will continue to educate those who get these oils through articles on our website. These articles will be devoted to restoring God's Temple through prayer, fasting, diet and essential oils. This is my assignment for the Lord and I will do it to the best of my abilities.

CONCLUSION

Essential oils are not a substitute for Christ or the price He paid over sin, sickness and death. These oils are a specific tool designed for those who desire restoration in their minds and bodies.

These oils are constructed from the inspiration of the Holy Spirit and personal use. I will pray over each one until I feel His presence and breath over the mixture.

Many times in the services I wish I could pray and lay hands on each person individually. Unfortunately, time and facilities prevent that from happening, but not this time.

These oils can touch those I could not and with the same anointing.

Again I say unto you, that if two of you shall agree on earth as touching anything that they shall ask, it shall be done for them of my Father who is in heaven. Matthew 8:19

The Holy Spirit is our healer and He has given me authority over sickness and the same authority that is in my life will come on those who believe. God is no respecter of persons. The oils, as a result of their unique properties, will activate your faith and be a point of contact for our agreement.

Mark 6:13 And they cast out many demons, and anointed with oil many who were sick, and healed them.

This is my prayer for you:

Holy Spirit I know you hear me because you have instructed me to provide your Body with these tools, in order for you to intervene and answer their prayers.

I ask you to give me the wisdom to prepare the oils for each of those who desire your presence in their daily lives. Let this be the beginning of a revolutionary change in the health and well-being.

Father my heartbreaks for those whose bodies have been

destroyed through medicines and are perishing because they are too sick to hear your instructions. I ask you to allow these oils to change their body chemistry dramatically enough for them to experience the ecstasy of your presence and fulfill the call on their life.

In Christ Name AMEN
L. Emerson Ferrell

APPLICATION OF OILS

E ach of these oils has been designed through the direction of the Holy Spirit. The oils have been activated through prayer with the specific purpose to change the conditions of the user. They are not inanimate objects but should be considered alive and capable of altering the physical and mental conditions of those who use them.

Essential oils are designed by God and contain His love and as such should be considered a spiritual bridge between your faith and Him. They will supply your cells with the spiritual frequencies necessary to provide health and healing. The detoxification process can be uncomfortable and even nauseating but it is required in most cases to "reset" the DNA in the cells to their proper conditions.

People often ask, "what will this oil do?" My response is what do you want it to do? The answer is not flippant because I know the power God has hidden inside His creation.

The very source of life is hidden inside the chemistry of plants. If the green plants did not exist on the earth neither would man.

They are the filters that transform carbon dioxide into oxygen and without that chemical reaction man could not live on planet earth.

Therefore, would it not make sense that God would use the life inside the plant to maintain the life of man? The symbiotic relationship is undeniable.

The application of the oils should be done in faith morning, noon and night without any reluctance or concerns.

I suggest inhaling and massaging the oils with thanksgiving even in the midst of pain. Changing our sensitivity to pain is one of the purposes of essential oils.

The attention to our many blessing with love and appreciation in conjunction with the oils will truly work miracles.

God created our bodies to work in harmony with each center and below is a list of some of the most important ones.

1. Integumentary System - skin, hair, nails, sense receptors, sweat glands, oil glands.

2. Skeletal System - bones, cartilage, joints.
3. Muscular System - muscles attached to bones.
4. Nervous System - brain, spinal cord, nerves, brain stem, sensory organs.

5. Endocrine System - pituitary gland, pineal gland, hypothalamus, thyroid gland, parathyroids, thymus, adrenals, pancreas, ovaries, testes.

6. Cardiovascular/Circulatory System - blood, heart, arteries, veins, blood vessels, capillaries.

7. Lymphatic/Immune System - lymph nodes, lymphatic vessels, thymus, spleen, lymph, tonsils.

8. Respiratory System - nose, pharynx, larynx, trachea, bronchi, lungs.

9. Urinary System - kidneys, ureters, bladder, urethra.

10. Reproductive System - (male) testes, vas deferens, urethra, prostate, penis, scrotum; (female) ovaries, uterus, uterine tubes, vagina, vulva, mammary glands.

11. Digestive System - mouth, pharynx, esophagus, stomach, intestines, rectum, anal canal, teeth, salivary glands, tongue, liver, gallbladder, pancreas, appendix.

These are a few of the oils that have been used according to centers: (Note: the oils are alive. The Holy Spirit will activate the oils you have to meet the needs you have because faith is stronger than formulas)

12. Integumentary System - Lavender, Rosewood, Cedarwood, Menthol, Myrrh, Helichrysum, Frankincense, Peppermint, Lemon, Ylang Ylang, Palmarosa, Orange, Eucalyptus.

13. Skeletal System - Fennel, Cedarwood, Rose, Thyme, Oregano, Wintergreen, Peppermint, clove, Melissa, Spruce, Hyssop, Citronella, Orange, Eucalyptus.

14. Muscular System - Frankincense, Peppermint, Orange, Clove, Wintergreen, Tea Tree, Spearmint, Myrrh, Lavender, Palmarosa, Spruce, Cedarwood, Hyssop.

15. Nervous System - Lavender, Frankincense, Spikenard, Melissa, Myrrh, Peppermint, Clove, Wintergreen, Menthol, Endocrine System - Oregano, Thyme, Spikenard, Grapefruit, Citronella, Frankincense, Myrrh, Lavender, Clove.

16. Cardiovascular/Circulatory System - Menthol, Lavender, Lemon, Orange, Wintergreen, Ylang Ylang, Marjoram, Fennel, Rosewood, Cedarwood, Rose, Citronella.

17. Lymphatic/Immune System - Helichrysum, Tangerine, Lemon, Frankincense, Orange, Myrrh, Clove, Lavender, Grapefruit.

18. Respiratory System - Wintergreen, Lavender, Peppermint, Frankincense, Clove, Helichrysum, Spearmint, Thyme.

19. Urinary System - Myrrh, Tangerine, Wintergreen, Helichrysum, Clove.

20. Reproductive System - Ylang Ylang, Frankincense, Lavender, Myrrh, Orange,

21. Digestive System - Peppermint, Spearmint, Lemon, Tangerine, Frankincense, Orange, Clove, Ylang Ylang, Thyme

ALL OF THE ABOVE OILS ARE USED IN MY BLENDS AND MIXTURES. THOSE WITH THE HIGHEST FREQUENCIES ARE THE MOST OFTEN USED IN MY OILS.

The trillions of cells inside our bodies individually respond to a specific frequency designed to regenerate healthy cell growth and development. God preprogrammed the essential oils with compound resonating frequencies that can reset corrupted cells at the DNA level back to their original frequency of health.

The active ingredients in essential oils are constantly evolving from harvest to harvest to combat diseases. Antibiotics created in laboratories are unable to evolve and basically serve to make future strains of bacteria stronger.

GENERAL DIRECTIONS

Each of the essential oils can be used with the confidence and assurance that nothing inside the bottle is toxic or harmful.

METHODS OF APPLICATION

1. Drip one or more drops into the palm of your hands. Use your fingers to rotate the oil clockwise in your hand then apply it to your feet, arms, hands, back, legs, neck and shoulders. The essential oils are blended with "carrier" oils that are either jojoba or almond oil. These carrier oils increase the shelf life of the essential oil and slow the absorption rate into the skin.

2. For inhalation drip the oil into your palms and rub them together vigorously clockwise. Then cup your hands over your nose and breathe.

The higher frequency oils should be inhaled often and frequently to change the mental attitude and increase awareness of the Holy Spirit.

The middle to lower frequency oils should be applied to areas of the body in pain. Do not hesitate to use small drops in coffee and tea.

These beverages reduce our frequencies 15 to 25 MhZ. The immediate use of essential oils is effective in returning our frequencies to their normal ranges.

Negative thoughts also lower the body's frequencies but inhalation can quickly returns the system back to normal.

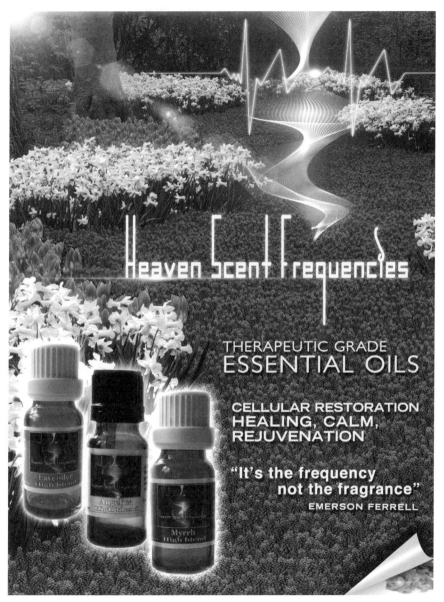

For orders, visit us at www.anamendezferrell.com or call us at 904.834.2447

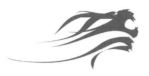

Ana Méndez Ferrell, INC.

Visit our online store at

www.anamendezferrell.com

Write to: Ana Méndez Ferrell, Inc.
P. O. Box 141
Ponte Vedra, FL 32004-0141
United States of America

Email: store@anamendezferrell.com

Like us on **FACEBOOK** or watch us on **YOUTUBE**

www.facebook.com/EmersonFerrell

www.youtube.com/Voiceofthelight

Recommended Books
L. Emerson Ferrell

-Quantum Fasting, Food for Thought

-Immersed in Him

-Becoming The Master's Key

-Supernatural Believing, Christ Conscious

About the author of *"The Breath of God Over Essentials Oils"*

L. Emerson is also the author of *"Supernatural Believing Christ Conscious," "Becoming the Master's Key," "Immersed in Him", and "Quantum Fasting, Food for Thought"* as well as, a profound worshipper and gifted artist. The Lord uses him in the prophetic to set captives free and establish God's Kingdom throughout the world.

L. Emerson Ferrell currently ministers with his wife Ana Méndez Ferrell. Together they train thousands of people on the reality of the spiritual realm and its power over the physical circumstances.